ACTIVATE CANNABIS FOR BEGINNERS

Decarboxylation of cannabis for beginners

Rüdiger Klos-Neumann

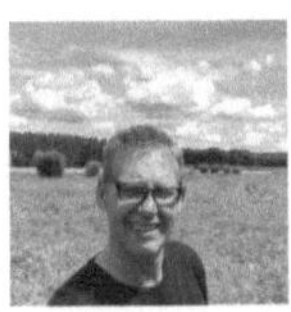

FOREWORD

This guidebook should not be missing from any well-stocked kitchen and home pharmacy. It provides the reader with valuable information on the responsible use of cannabis as a medicine and stimulant. This requires that the reader learns how to process the plant in order to make the best use of the active ingredients. In addition to the basics of use and further processing, there are examples of dosage for beginners. Recipes for the production of cannabis butter, oils, sugar and much more complete this easy-to-understand guide.

Cannabis is a spice with a special effect. There are hundreds of cannabis varieties. They differ in smell, taste and effect. In the kitchen, cannabis can be used like other herbs or spices to give food and drinks an extraordinary taste with a special effect. This knowledge is not new and has been used around the globe for thousands of years. A hundred years ago, cannabis was still part of our food chain. Cannabis is a very intense spice, so that even a few grams are enough to achieve the desired effect.

However, if you take too much cannabis, it can become unpalatable and the effect can be devastating. If the temperatures during processing are too high or too low, there will be no effect.

Caution: The use of cannabis as a medicine or stimulant may not be permitted in your country. Please inform yourself about the

current legal situation in order to avoid criminal prosecution.

1. WHY DOES CANNABIS NEED TO BE ACTIVATED?

The flavours and active ingredients are on the cannabis plant. If I were to eat fresh cannabis, the taste would be very intense, but there would be very little to no effect. It is only through heating that the active ingredients are activated so that the body can absorb them.

The activation of cannabis is also called decarboxylation. Some readers may only be familiar with cannabis in the form of a rolled cigarette (joint). The effect is known to come from combustion, where most of the flavours are lost and only about 15% of the active ingredients are absorbed. The effect lasts, depending on the variety, for a few hours until the "normal" state returns. When cannabis is ingested orally, the effect can be up to ten times stronger than when it is smoked. The effect is much more intense and can last 4-8 hours.

2. HOW TO ACTIVATE CANNABIS?

There are several methods to activate the active ingredients of cannabis. In the following chapters, water bath and oven activation will be explained in detail. Whether you want to use cannabis flowers, hashish or extracts, all products must be activated beforehand, so that the effect can begin with the oral intake. Which method is most suitable ultimately depends on the further processing of the activated cannabis.

For example, if you want to make a salad dressing, the taste should be in the foreground, in addition to the effect, and it is recommended to activate in a water bath. If it must go fast and only the effect is desired, one activates the cannabis in the oven.
Note: Good taste and effect there is in the activation in the water bath The needs, however, more time than in the oven and has less taste with the same effect!

3. WHAT TEMPERATURES MUST BE OBSERVED?

The right temperature and time are crucial for a good decarboxylation of cannabis products. Cannabis strains have different active ingredients (THC, CBD, CBG, CBN, etc.) and flavors that are activated from 80-150 degrees. For the activation we use best 100-120 degrees.

It should be noted that already at 155 degrees the THC active ingredient evaporates, which can be an essential component of the desired effect. When decarboxylating, one should always make sure to obtain as many active ingredients as possible, as these result in the interaction of the optimal effect. If you want to learn more about this, I recommend reading about the Entourage effect.

Note: At low temperature, the activation takes longer, but more flavors are retained. At high temperature, many flavors are lost, but the activation is faster!

4. DOSING GUIDE FOR FOOD CONTAINING CANNABIS

The effect of cannabis is different for each person. Those who have never tried cannabis products before will probably have a low tolerance. This means that even the smallest amounts of activated cannabis can have a very strong effect on the person.

Regular cannabis users, on the other hand, have a much higher tolerance. One should slowly approach the personally optimal dosage. Cannabis from unknown origin and active ingredient content should not be processed at all. It could be contaminated with harmful substances that are still present even after activation.

Always start with the lowest recommended dose. If necessary, increase the dose gradually, by 1 or 2 mg per dose, to find the optimal dose for you.

The content per dose:
1 mg - 2.5 mg THC

What to expect?

- Mild relief from pain, stress, anxiety, and other symptoms.
- Improved focus and creativity

Who is it suitable for?
- First-time users
- micro-dosers

The content per dose:
2.5 mg - 15 mg THC

What to expect?
- Greater symptom relief
- Euphoria
- May impair coordination and alter cognition.

Who is it suitable for?
- Patients with persistent problems
- Restless sleepers/insomnia.

The content per dose:
15 mg - 30 mg THC

What to expect?
- Strong euphoria or adverse effects in unaccustomed consumers
- May impair coordination and alter cognition

Who is it suitable for?
- Experienced consumers
- Medical patients with developed tolerances
- For experienced consumers who suffer from sleep problems.

The content per dose:
30 mg - 50 mg THC

What to expect?
- Very strong euphoria in unfamiliar consumers
- Likely to impair coordination and alter cognition

Who is it suitable for?
- Consumers who have poor absorption of cannabinoids
- People with significant tolerance to THC.

The content per dose:
50 - 100 mg THC

What to expect?
- May cause extreme side effects such as heart palpitations, nau-
sea, and pain
- May very likely impair coordination and alter cognition

Who is it suitable for?
- Only suitable for those experienced with cannabis - Patients
with cancer, inflammatory conditions, or conditions requiring
high doses

**Note: Never give someone activated cannabis without their
knowledge without first informing them of the possible effects.
It is true that to date no person has been proven to have died
from the use of cannabis. Nevertheless, it must be used respon-
sibly. Cannabis can, under certain circumstances, influence the
effect of medications positively as well as negatively. Too high a
dosage can lead to nausea, circulatory problems and heart palpi-**

tations.

5. PAINKILLER - CANNABIS AS MEDICINE

Cannabis is used internationally for a variety of conditions. The following is a list of diseases for which cannabis has been helpful as a medicine. Studies and further information in various languages can also be found on the Internet at www.cannabis-med.org.

Common:
- chronic pain
- multiple sclerosis
- Tourette's syndrome
- depressive disorders - ADHD.

Also:
- Allergic diathesis
- Anxiety disorder
- Loss of appetite and emaciation
- Arm plexus paresis
- Osteoarthritis

- Asthma
- Autism
- Barrett's esophagus
- Bladder spasms
- Blepharospasm
- Borderline disorder
- Lyme disease
- Chronic polyarthritis
- Chronic fatigue syndrome
- Pain syndrome after polytrauma
- Chronic spinal syndrome
- Cluster headaches
- Ulcerative colitis
- Epilepsy
- Failed-back surgery syndrome
- Fibromyalgia
- Hereditary motor-sensitive neuropathy with pain and spasm
- HIV infection
- Cervical and lumbar spine syndrome
- Hyperhidrosis syndrome Syndrome
- Hyperhidrosis
- Headache
- Lumbargia
- Lupus erythematosus
- Migraine accompagnée
- Migraine
- Mitochondropathy
- Bekhterev's disease
- Crohn's disease
- Scheuermann's disease
- Still's disease
- Sudeck's disease
- Neurodermatitis
- Paroxysmal nonkinesiogenic dyskinesia (PNKD) - Polyneuropathy
- Posner-Schlossmann

- Posttraumatic Stress Disorder
- Psoriasis
- Irritable Bowel Disease
- Rheumatism (rheumatoid arthritis)
- Sarcoidosis
- Sleep Disorders
- Painful Spasticity in Syringomyelia
- Systemic systemic scleroderma
- tetraspasticity after infantile cerebral palsy
- thalamus syndrome
- thrombangitis obliterans
- tics
- tinnitus
- trichotillomania
- urticaria of unknown origin
- cervicobrachialgia
- consequences of cranial brain trauma
- obsessive-compulsive disorder

Note: Cannabis can be a stimulant and painkiller at the same time. It depends on the dose!

6. ACTIVATE CANNABIS IN THE OVEN

Activating cannabis in the oven is a quick way to make the active ingredients available. It should be noted that when activating in the oven, it is possible that the whole apartment will smell of cannabis. What is needed: - Oven - Heat-resistant container made of glass, ceramic or metal, if possible with a lid - Cannabis of your choice (flowers, hashish, extract)

Steps:
1. Preheat the oven to 100 degrees.
2. Coarsely chop the cannabis flowers, remove the stems and fill the jar no more than halfway.
3. Heat the cannabis in the jar for 10 minutes at 100 degrees in the oven.
4. After 10 minutes, close the jar with a lid or aluminum foil.
5. Leave the jar in the oven at 115 degrees for 60 minutes
6. Remove the jar from the oven and allow to cool unopened
7. The activated cannabis can then be consumed directly or processed further.

Hash or extracts can be added directly to the jar. Allow these to remain in the sealed jar in the oven at 115 degrees for about 60 minutes. In the case of extracts, it is very easy to determine when activation is complete. If you observe the activation process in the oven, you can see how the extract forms small bubbles. After a good hour, no more bubbles form and the activation is complete.

7. ACTIVATE CANNABIS IN WATER BATH

Activating cannabis in a water bath is a low odor and active ingredient preserving method to activate it. However, it is also a bit more control-consuming than the oven method.   What is needed: - Stove - Pot - Heat resistant glass jar with lid or heat resistant vacuum bag to seal - Cannabis of choice (flower, hashish, extract).

Steps:
1. Fill the pot half full with water.
2. Roughly crush the cannabis flowers, remove the stalks, fill the jar up to a maximum of half and seal it. **3.** Place the cannabis in the jar in the water bath and boil for 90 minutes. Do not allow to boil unattended and occasionally refill with hot water. Alternatively, the cannabis can be placed in a heat-resistant vacuum bag and sealed, then activated directly into the water bath for 90 minutes.
4. Remove the jar/vacuum bag from the water bath and allow to cool unopened
5. Ready the activated cannabis for consumption or further processing.

Hash or extracts can be added directly to the jar or vacuum bag.

These are also activated for 90 minutes in a boiling water bath.

Tip: To ensure that the jar floats and does not touch the bottom of the pot, you can place a metal cookie cutter on the bottom of the pot, for example. Otherwise, air bubbles will form under the jar and it will begin to move back and forth noisily in the pot.

8. CANNABIS BUTTER

To make cannabis butter, there are different methods, all of which lead to the goal. The preparation is about combining the best possible taste and effect. Optimal results are obtained when the cannabis has been activated beforehand. This saves time and guarantees the effect. Since the active ingredients and flavors of the plant are fat soluble, the butter should have a high fat content.

For all the following methods, it is recommended to clarify the butter before further processing. To do this, simply melt the butter at a low temperature and then place it in the refrigerator or freezer to harden again. For portioning, it is important to note that with a package of butter of 250 g, only 200 g remain after clarifying. The less water there is in the butter, the longer the shelf life.

Attention: As a beginner without previous experience with cannabis it is recommended to start with a low dosage. Per serving of cannabis butter this would be 0.25 g cannabis flowers, 0.1 g hashish, 0.05 g cannabis extract.

Initial dosages examples: Assuming that each ready-to-eat serving of cannabis butter weighs 10 grams, the following mixing ratio comes into question:

- 200 grams of clarified butter mixed with 5 grams of cannabis flowers
- 200 grams of clarified butter mixed with 2 grams of hashish
- 200 grams of clarified butter mixed with 1 gram of cannabis extract.

Method 1 - What is needed:
- Stove
- Pot
- Metal or glass bowl that can be placed on the pot
- Strainer
- Cellulose cloth, or coffee or tea filter
- Butter of choice
- Fine scale
- Cannabis of choice (flowers, hashish, extract).

Steps:
1. Fill the pot halfway with water and place the bowl on top. Now put the desired amount of activated cannabis and butter together in a bowl and heat it. Leave the cannabis butter mixture on the water bath for a good 2 hours, stirring occasionally. Do not allow to boil unattended and occasionally add hot water.
2. Then run the mixture through a sieve to remove most of the plant matter. To further enhance the butter, it can be passed luke-warm through a cellulose cloth or coffee filter.
3. To portion the butter, it can be placed in an ice cube mold or ice cube bag. This way each portion contains the same amount of active ingredients.

Method 2 - What is needed:
- Stove
- Pot
- Strainer
- Coffee or tea filter
- Butter as desired
- Heat resistant glass jar with lid or heat resistant vacuum bag to seal
- Cannabis as desired (flower, hashish, extract)

- Fine scale.

Steps:
1. Put the butter and the previously activated cannabis in a sealable jar.
2. Heat a pot of water and boil the jar with the cannabis-butter mixture in the water bath for 2 hours. Do not allow to boil unattended and occasionally add hot water. The jar contents should be surrounded by water. Alternatively, the cannabis butter mixture can be placed in a heat-resistant vacuum bag and sealed. Then simmer the vacuum bags in a water bath for 2 hours.
3. Remove the jar or vacuum bag from the water bath and allow to cool slightly unopened.
4. Then run the mixture through a sieve to remove most of the plant matter. To further enhance the butter, it can be passed lukewarm through a cellulose cloth or coffee filter. 6. To portion the butter, it can be placed in an ice cube mold or ice cube bag. This way, each portion contains the same amount of active ingredients.

Method 3 - What is needed:
- Rice stove
- Strainer
- Coffee or tea filter
- Butter of your choice
- Cannabis of your choice (flower, hash, extract)
- Fine scale.

Steps:
1. Put the butter and the previously activated cannabis directly into the rice stove and simmer on the lowest setting for 2-4 hours, stirring regularly.
2. At the end of the time, pass the mixture through a sieve to remove most of the plant parts. To make the butter even finer, it can be passed lukewarm through a cellulose cloth or coffee filter.
3. To portion the butter, it can be placed in an ice cube mold or ice

cube bag. This way each portion contains the same amount of active ingredients.

Activated hash or extracts can be placed directly into a jar or vacuum bag with the butter. These concentrated active ingredients dissolve most quickly in the butter. Already after 5-10 minutes the hashish or extract should have dissolved.

Storage and shelf life of cannabis butter:
To preserve the taste and effect of cannabis butter for a long time, it should be stored covered in the refrigerator. As a rule, it can then be kept for 10-14 days. Alternatively, cannabis butter can be frozen in portions for up to 3 months.

Note: There is another method where cannabis and butter are cooked directly with water in a pot. The big disadvantage here is the loss of flavors and reduced effect.

Note: It is recommended to make the butter with activated cannabis, because the temperature during the production is too low to ensure a good decarboxylation in time.

9. CANNABIS OILS

Theoretically, all cold-pressed oils can be used to dissolve the cannabis active ingredients. Whereby coconut oil, peanut oil and olive oil do not go rancid so quickly and are excellent carrier oils thanks to their particularly good bioavailability.

Starting dosages examples:
- 500 ml oil mixed with 10 g activated cannabis flowers - 500 ml oil mixed with 2.5 g activated hashish
- 500 ml oil mixed with 1 g activated extract.

Certainly not the fastest, but the best tasting method simply mix the desired oil with activated cannabis flowers, and pour into a sealable bottle. This store in a dark and cool place Regularly shake the bottle, so that the active ingredients are released from the plant material. After 3-4 weeks, the oil should have a good concentration of flavor and active ingredients. It can then be passed through a sieve with cellulose cloth.

Much faster is the method of heating activated cannabis flowers, hashish or extracts with the desired oil. For this method, you can also use a water bath with glass (1-2 hours) or vacuum bag (1 hour), as with cannabis butter. Likewise, the rice stove (1-2 hours) on the lowest setting offers a safe preparation option. In a pinch, the mixture can also be put directly into a pot and heated on the lowest setting for 1-2 hours. Regular stirring supports the process of transferring the flavor and active ingredients to the oil. As with honey, the temperature during preparation should not exceed 30 degrees.

Tip: *To season and refine dishes, simply put the cannabis oil in a spray dispenser.*

Storage and shelf life of cannabis oil: Store the cannabis oil in opaque containers, daylight destroys important ingredients and makes the oil rancid faster. If stored well, it should keep for 2-3 months after preparation.Close cannabis oils immediately after use to protect it from contamination.

10. CANNABIS HONEY

As already known, fat or alcohol is needed to separate the active ingredients from the plant. Therefore, honey itself can not dissolve the active ingredients. Nevertheless, there are some methods how to prepare cannabis honey. Mixing activated cannabis flowers with honey therefore does not make much sense. It is more recommended to refine the honey with cannabis extracts, highly concentrated oils or tinctures.

Starting dosages examples: If a portion of cannabis honey should correspond to a level teaspoon of 10 g, the following mixing ratio comes into question:
- 500 g honey mixed with 5 g activated hashish
- 500 g honey mixed with 2.5 g activated extract.

The simplest method is to heat honey and cannabis extract separately and then mix them. The temperature of 30 degrees should not be exceeded. In order for the cannabis to be optimally distributed in the honey, it is recommended to complete the process with a mixing rod.

If you do not have cannabis extract at hand, you can alternatively process cannabis coconut oil or cannabis tincture in the same way. To prevent the cannabis coconut oil from floating on the surface after mixing, it should be processed very well with the mixing rod. When mixing with an alcohol tincture, the alcohol will evaporate almost completely over time. Repeated stirring and regular opening of the honey jar favors this process.

Storage and shelf life: Honey in itself has an unlimited shelf life. From experience, the cannabis honey is consumed faster than expected.

Tip: *The cannabis honey is well suited for wound healing and has an anti-inflammatory effect both externally and internally.*

11. CANNABIS TINCTURE

An alcohol-based cannabis tincture can be produced quickly and simply. For this purpose, a preferably high percentage alcohol from 60% is needed to dissolve the flavor and active ingredients. Wine spirit with 96% alcohol is optimal, but it is NOT suitable for direct, undiluted consumption! To make it drinkable, the cannabis tincture is diluted in a mixing ratio of 1:5 (1 part cannabis tincture and 5 parts fruit juice/water). This gives 18-20% alcohol content in the mixed drink.

Starting dosages examples:
If a portion of cannabis tincture diluted 1:5 should correspond to 10 ml, the following mixing ratio comes into question:
- 500 ml of alcohol mixed with 10 g of activated cannabis flowers
- 500 ml of alcohol mixed with 2 g of activated hashish - 500 ml of alcohol mixed with 1 g of activated extract.

What is needed:
- Freezer
- Sealable jar, or cocktail shaker
- Strainer
- Pulp cloth or tea strainer

- Bottle with cap
- Activated cannabis flowers, hashish or extract.

Cannabis tincture preparation:

1. Put the activated cannabis in a freezer bag and freeze for 12 hours. Also freeze the spirit with bottle, sealable glass/cocktail shaker and strainer for 12 hours.

2. After 12 hours, mix the activated cannabis with the alcohol in the glass or cocktail shaker and shake vigorously for 3-4 minutes. This will cause the frozen flavors and active ingredients to separate from the plant material and transfer into the spirit of wine.

3. Now strain the cannabis tincture through the frozen sieve and then refine the liquid again through cellulose cloth or fine tea strainer.

Storage and Shelf Life:

Bottle cannabis tincture and label with safety instructions. Cannabis tincture can be stored at room temperature or in the refrigerator for 6-12 months.

Usage: *The diluted cannabis tincture can be used to refine hot and cold drinks, as well as seasoning food or marinades. There are no limits to the imagination.*

Note: <u>High-percentage ethyl alcohol undiluted can lead to significant damage to health and even death.</u>

12. CANNABIS SALT & SUGAR

Cannabis can be used like rosemary, tyhmian or other herbs for seasoning food. Thus, one should always have a salt mill filled with activated cannabis and coarse sea salt in the spice rack. If you only want to transfer the taste and active ingredients to the salt, the cannabis tincture is the key to success.

Preparation Cannabis Salt:
Spread 500 g of salt on a clean baking sheet. Now spread 100 ml of cannabis tincture over it. Mix the mixture well and then smooth the mixture on the baking sheet and cover it with a kitchen towel. Depending on the room temperature, it takes a few days for the alcohol to evaporate and a salt plate to remain on the baking sheet. You can accelerate the process in the oven with circulating air at the lowest temperature. After just over an hour the alcohol has evaporated. Attention always ventilate well so that there is no harmful concentration of alcohol in the room air. Crush the cannabis salt plate with your hands and put it into a salt mill or shaker.

Preparation Cannabis Sugar:
Spread 500 g of sugar on a clean baking sheet. Now spread 100 ml of cannabis tincture over it. Mix the mixture well and then

smooth the mixture on the baking sheet and cover with a kitchen towel. Depending on the room temperature, it takes a few days for the alcohol to evaporate and a sugar slab to remaan on the baking sheet. You can accelerate the process in the oven with circulating air at the lowest temperature. After just over an hour the alcohol has evaporated. Attention always ventilate well so that no harmful alcohol concentration can occur in the room air. Crush the cannabis sugar slab with your hands and put it into a container or shaker. In a blender, the cannabis sugar can also be crushed into fine cannabis powdered sugar.

Storage and shelf life:
At room temperature, in a closed container store dry, salt and sugar are 2-3 months usable until the active ingredients have degraded.

13. CANNABIS CHOCOLATE

Cannabis chocolate is a delicious snack for in between or well suited to refine other dishes. For this purpose, the personal favorite can be used as well as commercially available couverture. When processing chocolate, you need to pay attention to two things. First, the temperature should not exceed 50 ° C when melting and secondly, make sure that no water gets into the chocolate mass. Even a small amount of water can cause the mass to clump. If the chocolate mass is heated too much, it begins to harden and must be diluted with butter, cream or oil. However, this changes the melting point of the chocolate mass. This then becomes less solid in the end result and takes a little longer to harden and should be included in the calculation.

When tempering by hand, the chocolate is first completely melted, usually by heating it to a temperature of 45 to 50 °C in a water bath.

Starting dosages Examples:
If a portion of cannabis chocolate is to be equivalent to 20 g, the following mixing ratio is possible:
- 200 g of chocolate mixed with 10 ml of activated cannabis oil
- 200 ml of chocolate mixed with 2 g of activated hashish

- 200 ml of chocolate mixed with 1 g of activated extract.

What is needed:
- Stove
- Pot
- Metal or glass bowl that can be placed on the pot
- Whisk
- Dough scraper
- Baking paper or aluminum foil
- Chocolate
- Scale
- Activated cannabis oil, hashish or extract

Steps:
1. Fill the pot halfway with water and place the bowl on top. Now roughly chop the chocolate and add it to the bowl. Heat the water bath on low heat and melt the chocolate.
2. Now remove the liquid chocolate mass from the stove and stir in the desired amount of activated cannabis oil, hashish or extract with a whisk until everything has mixed with the chocolate mass.
3. For portioning, the chocolate mass can be placed in a home-made mold made of baking paper or aluminum foil. Should the cannabis chocolate be placed in the refrigerator to cool, it could tarnish white and become unsightly. At room temperature, it takes a little longer for the chocolate mixture to harden. Weigh the cannabis chocolate whole first, then portion it into 20g pieces.

Storage and Shelf Life:
It is best to store the cannabis chocolate in an airtight container, away from intense odors, moisture and strong light. The higher the cocoa content, the longer the shelf life. While dark chocolate will keep for up to 24 months and milk chocolate for up to 18 months, white chocolate will keep for approximately 12 months.

Tips:
Cannabis chocolate can be refined with nuts, cornflakes or fruit pieces, for example. However, this reduces the shelf life considerably. Of course, the cannabis chocolate can be melted again to make cannabis chocolate fruit or an ice cream topping. Cookies and pastries can be super decorated with it, or may it rather be a cannabis chocolate muffin. If you prefer cakes, you can bake with the cannabis chocolate or make delicious creams.

Note: Avoid water getting into the chocolate mass and make sure not to heat it above 50 °C.

14. CANNABIS EGGNOG

In our village we always have an eggnog or two with our coffee. This recipe is quite simple and can be refined in different ways with activated cannabis products. You have the choice to enrich the active ingredients either with cannabis sugar and or cannabis tincture. It is virtually a part of the regular ingredients replaced by cannabis products.

Initial dosages examples:
If a glass should correspond to 20 ml, the following mixing ratio comes into question:
- 500 ml eggnog mixed with 20 ml activated cannabis tincture
- 500 ml eggnog mixed with 50 g activated cannabis sugar.

What is needed:
- Mixing bowl
- Bowl
- Cup
- Hand mixer or food processor
- Strainer

- Funnel
- Scale
- Bottles with cap
- Activated cannabis sugar, or cannabis tincture.

Ingredients:
- 500 ml Doppelkorn 38 %
- 240 g sugar
- 2 x canned milk with 12% fat
- 10 egg yolks
- 2 packets vanilla sugar

Steps:
1. Separate the yolks from the whites and put them in a cup.
2. Put all the ingredients in the mixing bowl in order and mix for 5-10 minutes.
3. Strain the cannabis egg liqueur through a sieve into the second bowl.
4. With the help of the funnel, bottle the eggnog and store it in the refrigerator.
5. the longer the eggnog is stored, the more viscous the consistency becomes.

Storage and shelf life:
When stored in the refrigerator, Cannbis eggnog should keep for 6-12 MOnate.

15. CANNABIS COOKIES

This recipe is quite simple and can be refined in different ways with activated cannabis products. You can choose to enrich the active ingredients with either cannabis sugar or cannabis butter. It is virtually a part of the regular ingredients replaced by cannabis products.

Starting dosages examples:
On the amount of dough in the recipe, the following dosage comes into question:
- 200 g activated cannabis butter
- 150 g activated cannabis sugar

What you need:
- Oven
- Baking trays
- Baking paper
- Cookie cutters

- Rolling pin
- Mixing bowl
- Sieve
- Scales
- Metal tins or jars for storage
- Activated cannabis sugar and/or cannabis butter

Ingredients:
- 500 g flour
- 250 g sugar
- 250 g butter
- 2 eggs
- 2 packets vanilla sugar
- ½ packet baking powder
- 1 pinch of salt.

Steps:
1. Sift the flour into the mixing bowl and then add the rest of the ingredients.
2. knead the mixture vigorously until a uniform dough is formed. If the dough still sticks to your fingers, add a little more flour.
3. Cover the dough and place it in the refrigerator for about an hour.
4. Dust the work surface with a little flour and roll out half of the dough from the refrigerator evenly with a rolling pin.
5. Cut out the cookies with cookie cutters and place them on the baking tray 1-2 cm apart. Bake the cookies at 145 °C for 12-15 minutes until golden brown. Let the cookies cool down and roll out the remaining dough as before, cut out the cookies and bake. Once all the cookies have cooled completely, store in metal tins or sealable jars.

Storage and Shelf Life:
Stored dry at dew temperature, the cookies will keep for 3-4 months. Alternatively, the cookies can be frozen for 4-6 months.

16. COOKING AND BAKING WITH CANNABIS

With the knowledge from this guide of the methods, temperatures and times used in cannabis activation (decarboxalization), cannabis can be added to foods and beverages. With the presented cannabis base products such as cannabis butter, honey, oils, salt & sugar, a variety of dishes can be used in the preparation or for seasoning. It is always important to ensure that the cannabis products produced are not exposed to high temperatures, short or long term. This would only lead to the loss of flavor and active ingredients. Recipes containing sugar, oil, butter or alcohol are simply to be replaced in part or completely by the presented cannabis products.

Good luck and happy cooking!

ABOUT THE AUTHOR

Rüdiger Klos-Neumann

For more than 25 years, the family father Rüdiger Klos-Neumann has been suffering from one of the most painful illnesses people can suffer from. Cluster headache, also known as suicide headache, is still an incurable disease that leads to suicide in 55% of affected patients. It was only with cannabis therapy that cluster headache at-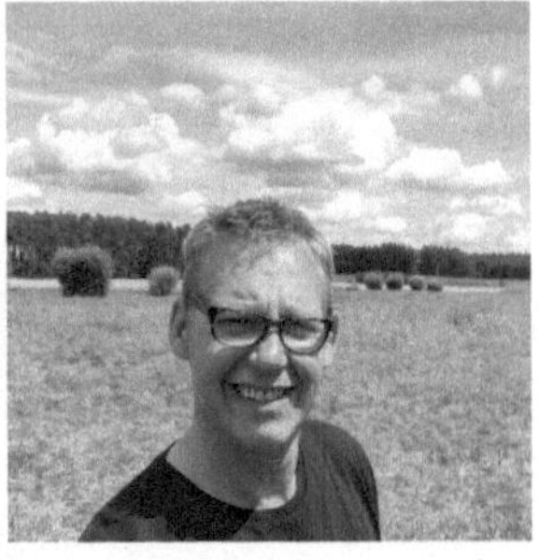tacks could be reduced in duration, intensity and repetition to a pain tolerable level. Among other things, this also repeatedly led to the restoration of employment. Without cannabis medication, Rüdiger Klos-Neumann suffers 4-6 cluster attacks daily, each lasting about 90 minutes, with a pain intensity of 8-9 on the pain scale. With cannabis therapy, he suffers 2-3 cluster attacks, each lasting 5-20 minutes, with a pain intensity of 2-4. Meanwhile, Rüdiger Klos-Neumann has six years of daily therapy experience with cannabis as medicine. As a trained chef, he also contributes his experience in the use of cannabis in the kitchen. He draws on his own experiences from cannabis therapy, as well as from travels to countries where cannabis is used legally as a medicine as well as a stimulant.

BOOKS BY THIS AUTHOR

We Ed 2050 - Aussicht Auf Bessere Zeiten

Im Jahr 2020 wurde der soziale Verfall unserer Gesellschaft massiv beschleunigt. Eine Pandemie veranlasste die Politik, die Menschen auf der ganzen Welt über Jahre zu isolieren. Zwischenmenschliche Kommunikation und Interaktion waren nur noch digital möglich. Die Wirtschaft erschuf die perfekte virtuelle Realität, um den Konsum und vor allem die Konsumenten umfassend steuern zu können. Bis ein kosmisches Ereignis die Menschen auf der Erde stark dezimierte.

Milliardäre mit ihren Familien, die wussten was bevorstand, verließen frühzeitig die Erde, um einen neuen Planeten zu besiedeln. Unser Planet war jedoch nicht verloren und begann sich zu regenerieren. Die übrig gebliebenen Menschen lebten wieder im Einklang mit der Natur, während sich auf Titan dem Eismond die Neubesiedlung der Millions zum Desaster entwickelte